47 Homemade Natural Perfume Recipes

Floral, Earthy, Herbal, Sandalwood And Other Fragrances

EMILY FISHER

ISBN-13:978-1983929717

ISBN-10:1983929719

DEDICATION

Phil & Merry, Love You Much!

TABLE OF CONTENT

INTRODUCTION 1

Why Wear Perfumes? 1

Why Homemade Perfumes? 3

Essential Oils, Alcohol and Your Fragrance 5

Perfume Tips To Remember 7

Perfume Making- Getting Started 10

HERBAL AND EARTHY SCENTS RECIPES 13

Woodland Perfume 13

Lavender Vanilla Perfume..................................... 14

Citrus Lavender Solid Perfume 15

Hungary Flower Perfume...................................... 16

Lavender Chamomile Perfume 17

Sandalwood Jojoba Perfume 18

Sandalwood Bergamot Perfume 19

Midnight Garden Perfume..................................... 20

Cucumber Aloe Perfume 21

Tropical Body Perfume 22

FLORAL RECIPES 25

Passionate Scent Perfume 25

Inspiring Floral Scent Perfume.............................. 26

Glittery And Dazzling Floral Scent Perfume 27

Floral Scent of love Perfume 29

Enchanted Floral Scented Perfume 30

Lavender Scented Solid Perfume............................ 31

Rose petals Scented Solid Perfume 33

Sweet Vanilla Scented Perfume............................. 34

Ylang ylang and lavender Scented Perfume 36

Walk In the Garden Floral Perfume 37

Cypress And Rosemary Scented Perfume 39

Chamomile And Valerian Scented Perfume 40

Cassis And Bergamot Scented Perfume 42

Musk, Sandalwood And Frankincense Scented
Perfume 43

Assorted Essential Oils Scented Perfume 45

Lavender Scented Perfume 46

Lilac Scented Perfume 47

Rose Scented Perfume...................................... 49

Orange Blossoms Scented Perfume 50

Orange and Cinnamon Scented Perfume 51

Rose, Chamomile and Lavender Scented Perfume .. 53

Foresty Scented Perfume 54

Summer Scent Perfume..................................... 55

Sweet Floral Scent Perfume 57

Gorgeous Floral Scented Perfume 58

MIXED PERFUME RECIPES 61

Sweet Flowery Perfume Recipe 61

Refreshing Woody Body Mist 62

Refreshing Citrus Mist 63

Refreshing Lavender And Vanilla Mist....................... 64

Flowery Scent 66

Fresh Peppermint And Vanilla Perfume 67

Sandalwood And Cassis Perfume 68

Relaxing Chamomile and Jasmine Perfume.............. 69

Refreshing Lemon Grass and Geranium Perfume 70

Refreshing Oriental Scent... 71

SCENTED WATERS.. 73

Orange Water 73

Rose Water 74

Lavender Water 75

Rosemary Water 76

INTRODUCTION

Why Wear Perfumes?

The word, perfume comes from a Latin word that means scented mixtures. Historically, the Egyptians were the first to incorporate the use of perfumes into their culture and religious ceremonies. For instance, cassia and myrrh (a form of cinnamon) was used in mummifying and embalming their dead bodies. Soon its usage spread to other nationalities like the Persians, the Greek and the Chinese.

However, in the 1900s, the advent of technology gave rise to the inclusion of synthetic ingredients as a substitute to natural perfume ingredients which were becoming scarcer. This led to mass production of perfumes and the product became available for everyone.

Also in this era, another perception of perfume was gradually introduced. In addition to the fragrance, other elements such as bottling, wrapping and advertising took priority. Perfumes began to be created as a fashion line supplement.

All these are introductory insights into how perfumes became an intricate part of our culture. Today, the wearing of perfume helps to boost self- confidence in both men and women. For a lot of women, it makes them feel happy, feminine, confident and beautiful.

Perfume has a very strong emotional feel with the ability to shift moods. It has an appeal that is both empowering and ephemeral and creates an invisible armor long after the wearer leaves a room. It even provides a hint of the wearer's attributes and personality! One sniff of perfume can revive childhood memories, long-forgotten memories of events or any other pleasant ones, bringing up tender feelings links with such special moment.

Perfume wearing facilitates romance and the wonderful art of seduction. According to studies, women's sense of smell is much stronger than men. Studies also show that men who smell good are more likely to attract good looking women and vice versa. However, this is a debatable topic because more and more women these days are becoming increasingly aware of their need for personal satisfaction and pleasure.

Fragrances, which is the type of scent emitted from a perfume is also viewed as an indication of class, a status symbol. Since there are quite a lot of offensive smelling and cheap perfumes in the market, there are ladies who feel "rich"- financially well-off due to the type of perfume that they wear.

However, perfumes should also be moderately applied. Remember that less is more.

Why Homemade Perfumes?
Ok. Someone might say, with the plethora of perfumes in the market. Why do I need to make my own? There are several benefits of making your own perfume.

- Save money

Since perfumes have become part of a beauty item for us. We will continually spend money on them for as long as we live but when you make your own, you get to save a considerable amount. You get to use them for much longer time too.

- All natural

You are sure of the ingredients so no synthetic, dangerous chemicals on your delicate skin. Will it surprise you to hear that manufacturers protect their trade secret by not listing all chemical ingredients on labels? Substances which have been proven to cause allergy and disrupt hormones are usually concealed.

Additionally, quite a number of commercial products contain chemical fragrances of an ingredient such as the smell of Rose and not the actual ingredient (Rose) themselves.

- No fake purchases

It is estimated that about 15% of perfume products are fake. Apart from the fact that buying fakes is criminal, may put individuals out of jobs and deprive the original manufacturer of hard earned revenue, buying fakes could be detrimental to your health in many ways.

It may contain dangerous chemicals which when absorbed into the skin could cause dermatitis or irritation of some sort. Manufacturers of commercial perfume products may use inferior substitutes for instance acetyl cedrene, a chemical used in rubber and also plastic goat's urine may also be used as a stabilizer.

Purchasing fakes may cause allergy to people who have sensitive skins and get your favorite clothes stained as well.

- Cut through the clutter

Like me, we may be confused by the plethora of fragrances in the market, every one of them with outlandish and overwhelming names such as perfume, parfum, eau de colognes, eau de toilettes, Eau de parfum and the likes. Heck! The bottom-line is to have the right smell at the right time for the right occasion. Making your own guarantees you all that and less time is spent in making a decision.

Essential Oils, Alcohol and Your Fragrance

Essential oil is a major ingredient used in perfume making. Alcohol is another vital ingredient while fragrance is the scent of the perfume. It is important to thoroughly understand the role these three elements play.

A variety of essential oils are available. Sandalwood, vanilla, lavender, amber, bergamot, cedarwood and freesia are some of the stand-out ones but neroli (orange blossom), jasmine and rose are much more expensive than others.

Simple facts about essential oils:
- 50 pounds of Juniper berries turns out 1 pound of essential oil
- 80 pounds of rosemary turns out 1 pound of essential oil
- 100 pounds of coriander seeds produce 1 pound of essential oil
- 200 pounds of lemon zests (oils must be concentrated) generates 1 pound of essential oil
- Over 250 pounds of lavender flowers creates a pound of lavender oil

The level of essential oil composition in the product determines the kind of fragrance you will get. The fragrance determines how much the perfume will cost. Perfumes become more affordable when alcohol is added to it. Alcohol is added to perfume because as it evaporates, it diffuses the scent of your fragrance. This way, people around you easily know you are wearing a perfume.

A perfume's lasting power is dependent on the quantity of alcohol in it. The less alcohol it contains, the longer the fragrance. Usually, a fragrance stays for about 6-8 hours but this also depends on the type of skin that you have.

People with oily skin may be able to wear their perfumes for longer periods because the natural moisture of oily skin can hold in the fragrance so small quantities are released all through the day.

The amount of acidity in the skin also known as PH levels vary from one person to another. Individual PH levels determine how each ingredient contained in a fragrance will react with your body chemistry.

Perfume Tips To Remember

Tips To Choose the Perfect Scent

All fragrances are categorized by their family group e.g. Woody, Floral, Oceanic, Fruity, Spicy etc. People tend to remain with a particular smell family because it recreates pleasurable memories or it simply stimulates their olfactory receptors.

To select the right scent for you, first, you have to think of which scents you truly enjoy wearing. You can create a list as a start. From lilacs to clean laundry and freshly cut grass, choose whatever smells you like and put them on the list. This helps you to remember the scents you really like in order to create a perfume with the same type of notes.

Next, choose a fragrance that best represents your personality. If you are always on the go or a party person, you might want a scent which really attracts and will stay for a while. Choose a fresh, clean scent as opposed to something musky or spicy if you are type that wears little or no makeup and stays outdoors a lot. Also, go for a fragrance that lingers and goes with your assertive outlook on life if you love to get dressed and consider yourself glamorous.

Test the scents first. Before using a perfume, you might as well try the scent of the perfume.

Furthermore, you can also ask for your family and friends' opinion on what perfume might suit you. Ask them if the scent is just too strong for you, too dry or if it goes well with your personality. But over all, it would pretty much depend on what scent you like and what others might think about it.

Notes of Perfume Fragrances

Perfumes usually contain layers of fragrances commonly referred to as notes. A particular perfume can have several notes. It doesn't give out the same scent on your skin, on the test strip and even in the bottle.

Top notes give you the "first impression of the smell". It is the first scent you smell when you put the perfume which quickly evaporates. This may be lime, orange, peppermint, lemon and many more

The middle notes which appear right after the top notes are gone. It makes up the majority of the scent. Middle notes could be basil, lavender, marjoram, rosemary, etc

Base notes are richer and are not immediately perceived until you've been wearing a scent for about 20 - 30 minutes. It stays the longest on the skin and lingers after the middle notes. Depending on the type of perfume, the base note may last up to 24 hours depending on the perfume. Some samples of the base notes are sandalwood, patchouli, frankincense, cedarwood, etc.

Perfume Application Tips

Here are a few tips to make your perfume last all day:

- Since fragrances react with heat, your cologne should be applied to pulse points such as wrist, back of knees, cleavage and back of neck.
- The blood vessels nearest to your skin give off heat and act like little scent diffusers and as you wear your perfume all through the day; you will easily emit your signature scent
- Rubbing your wrist together crushes the scent.
- Be sure to apply perfume from bottom to top, spray at the ankles so that the scent will rise and linger throughout the day.

Tips To Keep Your Perfume Fresh

- Keep at room temperature. Exposing perfumes to excessively cold or hot temperatures could affect the balance of certain ingredients or perfume notes.
- Keep bottle tightly closed. This prevents the alcohol from evaporating too soon.
- Store in dark places. Avoid direct sunlight.
- May be kept in a box. A dresser drawer or closets are also ideal.
- Perfume in opaque or blue bottles usually last longer than in clear bottles.
- Spray perfume containers have longer shelf life because they are sealed and not exposed to air.

Perfume Making- Getting Started

Step 1: Ingredients

- Vodka or Everclear if available
- Essential oils, fragrance oils, infused oils
- Glycerin (available in pharmacies)
- Distilled or spring water

Others include:

- Glass bottles for the finished product in such as colored glass or reuse bottles.
- glass jar for the mixing of fragrance
- Measuring cup/spoons
- a dropper, funnel
- wrapping paper or aluminum foil if you making use of clear glass bottles
- and of course, a discerning nose.

Step 2

Sterilize the bottles and the jars especially if you are reusing them. Cleanliness is always a must you know. Everything must be sterile and neat.

Measure ¼ cup of the vodka you have prepared and pour it into the glass jar.

Using a dropper, add 25 drops of the essential oil you have prepared beforehand. Here is what you need to do: add a few drops every now and then, shake the jar, smell the mixture, and decide on whether to add more drops.

This is totally the fun part! You can experiments on different volumes of the alcohol and the essential oil. Mix, drop, smell and get whatever desirable scent you want! Be a chemist, my friend!

Once you have achieved the scent that already makes you happy, you have to let it age then. Store it in a dark and cool location for the minimum period of 48 hours or for a month, depending on your desire. This process will allow the different scents to really mix well and give off a strong scent. After the ageing process of the mixture, smell it and decide whether it is already perfect for you. If it is too weak, add more drops as you desire.

After achieving the scent you desire, the mixture now needs to be diluted. You need to add 2 tablespoons of the distilled water. If you want a perfume spray, then add more water. You can preserve the fragrance even more by adding 5 drops of glycerin.

You are almost finished! Using a funnel, pour the mixture into the glass bottles you have already prepared. For the clear bottles, use aluminum foil or any wrapping paper to cover the bottle. This is because the perfume needs to be kept away from the light or else it might go off.

Finally, if you are planning to do this homemade perfume for business, decorate the wrap, add a label to the bottle and voila! You might be in line with Victoria's Secret perfume next year!

HERBAL AND EARTHY SCENTS RECIPES

Woodland Perfume

Preparation time: 2 minutes

Cooking time: 0 minutes

Ready in: 1 hour

Servings: 1 perfume bottle

Ingredients:

4 drops of spruce essential oil

2 drops of organic fir needle essential oil

2 drops of organic cedar wood essential oil

1 drop of vetiver essential oil

1 drop of organic bergamot essential oil

1 teaspoon of organic jojoba oil

Directions:
1. Take a glass bottle and add all the essential oils in it. Mix the oils by rolling the bottle between the palms.
2. After the oils get really mixed, add jojoba oil in the bottle and roll the bottle again.
3. If you desire a strong perfume, you could also add some other essential oils.

4.   The perfume gets ready to use within an hour.

Lavender Vanilla Perfume

Preparation time: 10 minutes

Cooking time: 0 minutes

Ready in: Four to six weeks

Servings: 1 perfume bottle

Ingredients:

½ cup of vodka

2 tablespoon of glycerin

1 cup of dried lavender flowers

Vanilla beans

15 drops of lavender essential oil

10 drops of vanilla extract

Directions:
1.   Slice the vanilla beans with sharp knife. Add the beans and lavender flowers in a large jar and pour vodka in it. Close the lid of the jar tightly.
2.   Keep the jar as it is for seven days.
3.   After seven days, remove the beans and lavender flowers from the jar. Pour the remaining ingredients in the jar and stir them properly.

4. Keep the mixture closed for four to six weeks. After that, filter out the mixture with the help of paper filter and transfer the resultant product into a perfume bottle.

Citrus Lavender Solid Perfume

Preparation time: 5 minutes

Cooking time: 2 minutes

Ready in: 10 minutes

Servings: 1 perfume bottle

Ingredients:

2 teaspoons of beeswax

2 teaspoons of carrier oil such as almond or jojoba oil

12 drops of lemon essential oil

10-12 drops of orange essential oil

10-12 drops of bergamot essential oil

10-12 drops of lavender essential oil

½ ounce of old lip balm

Directions:

1. Combine all the essential oils in a cup and allow them to mix well.

2. Put beeswax in small saucepan and melt it on medium heat. Add the almond oil or jojoba oil along with melted beeswax and stir them well.
3. Turn off the heat and add the remaining essential oils in it. Mix them well.
4. Pour this mixture into container and keep it settled for 10 minutes.
5. Ready to use.

Hungary Flower Perfume

Preparation time: 5 minutes

Cooking time: 0 minutes

Ready in: 10 hours

Servings: 1 perfume bottle

Ingredients:

50 ml of ethyl alcohol

12 drops of lemon essential oil

5 drops of rose essential oil

2 drops of sage essential oil

30 drops of rosemary essential oil

5 drops of neroil essential oil

2 drops of mint essential oil

Directions:

1. Take a bottle and put all the essential oils and ethyl alcohol in it. Keep it like this for 10 hours.
2. Shake it well before using and store it in a cool and dry place.
3. It is best used for one month from the time of manufacturing.

Lavender Chamomile Perfume

Preparation time: 5 minutes

Cooking time: 0 minutes

Ready in: 15 hours

Servings: 1 perfume bottle

Ingredients:

2-3 tablespoons of vodka or ethyl alcohol

10 drops of chamomile essential oil

2 cups of mineral water

5 drops of lavender essential oil

12 drops of valerian essential oil

Directions:

1. Take an airtight container and add all the essential oils and water in it. Shake them well.
2. Mix them well and let it settle for about 15 hours.
3. Shake it well before using.
4. Store it in a cool and dry place.

Sandalwood Jojoba Perfume

Preparation time: 2 minutes

Cooking time: 0 minutes

Ready in: 12-15 hours

Servings: 1 perfume bottle

Ingredients:

5 drops of musk essential oil

2 full teaspoons of jojoba oil

4 drops of sandalwood essential oil

2-3 drops of fragrance oil or frankincense essential oil

Directions:

1. Take a glass bottle and put all the essential oils in it. Mix them well and close the bottle tightly.
2. Allow it to get settled for 12-15 hours.
3. Ready to use. Shake it well before using and try to store it in a cool and dry place.

Sandalwood Bergamot Perfume

Preparation time: 5 minutes

Cooking time: 0 minutes

Ready in: 12-15 hours

Servings: 1 perfume bottle

Ingredients:

2-3 tablespoons of ethyl alcohol or vodka

9-10 drops of fragrance oil or bergamot essential oil

2 cups of distilled water

5 drops of sandalwood oil or fragrance essential oil

10 drops of cassis essential oil

Directions:

1. Take an airtight container and pour all the ingredients in the container. Mix them properly.
2. Allow it to get settled for 12-15 hours.
3. Shake it well before using and store it in a cool and dry place.

Midnight Garden Perfume

Preparation time: 5 minutes

Cooking time: 0 minutes

Ready in: 48 to six weeks

Servings: 1 perfume bottle

Ingredients:

2 tablespoons of almond or jojoba oil

6 tablespoons of vodka

2 and ½ tablespoons of distilled water

15 drops of clove oil

6 drops of cedar wood oil

9 drops of lavender oil

Two bottles for curing and storing

Coffee filter

Funnel

Directions:

1. Add almond oil or jojoba oil in one of the bottles. Next, add all the essential oils drop by drop. Add vodka in the bottle and then shake the mixture for several minutes. Close the bottle tightly.
2. Keep it settled for 48 to 6 weeks. Add distilled water to the mixture and shake it well.

3. Place coffee filter in a funnel and transfer the mixture from the bottle to the other bottle, storing bottle.
4. Shake it well before use and store it in dark and cool place.

Cucumber Aloe Perfume

Preparation time: 2 minutes

Cooking time: 0 minutes

Ready in: 5 minutes

Servings: 1 perfume bottle

Ingredients:

1 cucumber

1 lemon

1 teaspoon of aloe Vera gel

1 tablespoon of rosewater

Directions:

1. Blend cucumber in a blender for about one minute. Strain the cucumber juice in a bowl with the help of cheese cloth or napkin.
2. Add the remaining ingredients into the bowl and mix them well.

3. Transfer the mixture into perfume bottle and you can also add distilled water into the bottle for diluting the mixture.
4. Store it in a refrigerator.
5. It should be consumed within one week.

Tropical Body Perfume

Preparation time: 5 minutes

Cooking time: 0 minutes

Ready in: 2 hours

Servings: 1 perfume bottle

Ingredients:

30 ml of distilled water

2 teaspoons of vanilla extract

1 teaspoon of vodka

1 tablespoon of glycerin

1 tablespoon of coconut oil

5 drops of grapefruit

15 drops of neroil essential oil

Directions:

1. Take distilled water in a bottle. Add the mixture of vanilla extract and vodka into it.

2. Add glycerin and coconut oil in the bottle. Mix them well.
3. Add the remaining essential oils in the bottle and shake them well.

Allow it to get settled for one or two hours. Shake it well before use

FLORAL RECIPES

Passionate Scent Perfume

Prep Time: 5 minutes
Cook Time: 0 minutes
Ready In: 1 week
Servings: approximately 1 small perfume bottle

Ingredients:

Ylang ylang essential oil (2 drops)

Vodka (300 ml)

Neroli essential oil (3 drops)

Passionflower essential oil (3 drops)

Directions:

1. Pour in the vodka on a glass bottle which will be the container of your perfume. The bottle can be colored or clear.
2. Mix in the essential oils.
3. Shake the mixture very well to make sure everything blends in.
4. Let the mixture settle for a week, in a dark, dry and cool place. Shake the bottle every now and then. Take note of the fact that the longer you let the perfume settle and rest, the stronger the scent will be so it depends on you how long you would want the perfume to sleep.

5. Try out the perfume you have created. Shake the bottle well before using the perfume. Rub it on your wrist and neck. Check for any allergic reactions upon the application of the perfume to make sure it is safe on the skin.

6. Enjoy your very own homemade floral perfume!

Inspiring Floral Scent Perfume

Prep Time: 5 minutes
Cook Time: 0 minutes
Ready In: 12 hours
Servings: 1 big perfume bottle

Ingredients:

Vodka (3 tablespoons)

Cypress essential oil (10 drops)

Saint John's wort essential oil (5 drops)

Rosemary essential oil (10 drops)

Distilled water (2 cups)

Directions:

1. Using a dropper, drip the essential oils into a glass bottle (colored or clear glass bottle will do).
2. Close the bottle.
3. Shake the bottle to mix all the essential oils.
4. Add the vodka and water to the mixture.
5. Shake the bottle once again to mix the oils.

6. Let the mixture settle for 12 hours, in a dark, dry and cool place. Shake the bottle every now and then. Take note that the more hours you let the perfume settle and rest, the stronger the scent will be so it all depends on how long you want the perfume to sleep.
7. Try out the perfume you have created. Shake the bottle well before using the perfume. Rub it on your wrist and neck. Check for any allergic reactions upon the application of the perfume to make sure it is safe on the skin.
8. Enjoy your very own homemade floral perfume!

Glittery And Dazzling Floral Scent Perfume

Prep Time: 5 minutes
Cook Time: 0 minutes
Ready In: 12 hours
Servings: 1 big perfume bottle

Ingredients:

> Very fine body glitters
> Vodka (3 tablespoons)
> Lavender essential oil (5 drops)
> Valerian essential oil (10 drops)
> Chamomile essential oil (10 drops)
> Distilled water (2 cups)

Directions:

1. Using a dropper, drip the essential oils into a glass bottle (colored or clear glass bottle will do).
2. Close the bottle.

3. Shake the bottle to mix all the essential oils.
4. Add the vodka and distilled water to the mixture.
5. Shake the bottle once again to mix everything well.
6. Lastly add the glitters and shake.
7. Let the mixture settle for 12 hours, in a dark, dry and cool place. Shake the bottle every now and then. Take note that the more hours you let the perfume settle and rest, the stronger the scent will be so it depends upon you how long you would want the perfume to sleep.
8. Try out the perfume you have created. Shake the bottle well before using the perfume. Rub it on your wrist and neck. Check for any allergic reactions upon the application of the perfume to make sure it is safe on the skin.
9. Enjoy your very own homemade floral perfume!

Floral Scent of love Perfume

Prep Time: 5 minutes

Cook Time: 0 minutes

Ready In: 1 week

Servings: 1 perfume bottle

Ingredients:

Vodka (300 ml)

Cedar wood essential oil (3 drops)

Vanilla essential oil (2 drops)

Bergamot essential oil (15 drops)

Sandalwood essential oil (3 drops)

Directions:

1. Using a dropper, drip the essential oils into a glass bottle (colored or clear glass bottle will do).
2. Close the bottle.
3. Shake the bottle to mix all the essential oils.
4. Add the vodka to the mixture.
5. Shake the bottle once again to mix everything well.
6. Let the mixture settle for 1 week hours, in a dark, dry and cool place. Shake the bottle every now and then. Take note that the longer you let the perfume settle and rest, the stronger the scent will be so it all depends on you how long you want the perfume to sleep.
7. Try out the perfume you have created. Shake the bottle well before using the perfume. Rub it on

your wrist and neck. Check for any allergic reactions upon the application of the perfume to make sure it is safe on the skin.

8. Enjoy your very own homemade floral perfume!

Enchanted Floral Scented Perfume

Prep Time: 5 minutes
Cook Time: 0 minutes
Ready In: 24 hours
Servings: 1 big perfume bottle

Ingredients:

Very fine body glitters
Vodka (3 tablespoons)
Peony essential oil (10 drops)
Everlasting essential oil (5 drops)
Sandalwood essential oil (10 drops)
Distilled water (2 cups)

Directions:

1. Using a dropper, drip the essential oils into a glass bottle (colored or clear glass bottle will do).
2. Close the bottle.
3. Shake the bottle to mix all the essential oils.
4. Add the vodka and distilled water to the mixture.
5. Shake the bottle once again to mix everything well.
6. Lastly add the glitters and shake.

7. Let the mixture settle for 24 hours, in a dark, dry and cool place. Shake the bottle every now and then. Take note that the more hours you let the perfume settle and rest, the stronger the scent will be so it all depends on you how long you would want the perfume to sleep.

8. Try out the perfume you have created. Shake the bottle well before using the perfume. Rub it on your wrist and neck. Check for any allergic reactions upon the application of the perfume to make sure it is safe on the skin.

9. Enjoy your very own homemade floral perfume!

Lavender Scented Solid Perfume

Prep Time: 5 minutes
Cook Time: 0 minutes
Ready In: 24 hours
Servings: 1 floral scented soap

Ingredients:

Lavender essential oil (2 tablespoons)

Distilled water (2 tablespoons)

Sweet almond oil (2 tablespoons and 1 teaspoon)

Grated beeswax (2 tablespoons)

Emulsifying Wax (1/4 teaspoon)

Stearic acid (1/4)

Directions:

1. Using a double boiler, melt the emulsifying wax and beeswax until it becomes smooth. (Microwaves should not be used during this process.)
2. Add the stearic acid, water and sweet almond oil.
3. Stir the mixture while heating in the boiler so that everything mixes well.
4. Remove from heat.
5. Add the lavender essential oil.
6. Pour the mixture into jar containers.
7. Let the mixture harden.
8. Enjoy your very own homemade floral solid perfume!

Rose petals Scented Solid Perfume

Prep Time: 5 minutes

Cook Time: 0 minutes

Ready In: 24 hours

Servings: 1 floral scented soap

Ingredients:

Rose essential oil (2 tablespoons)

Sandalwood essential oil (1 tablespoon)

Distilled water (2 tablespoons)

Sweet almond oil (2 tablespoons and 1 teaspoon)

Grated beeswax (2 tablespoons)

Emulsifying Wax (1/4 teaspoon)

Stearic acid (1/4)

Directions:

1. Using a double boiler, melt the emulsifying wax and beeswax until it becomes smooth. (Microwaves should not be used during this process.)
2. Add the stearic acid, water and sweet almond oil.
3. Stir the mixture while heating in the boiler so that everything mixes well.
4. Remove from heat.
5. Add the sandalwood essential oil.

6. Stir the mixture.
7. Add the rose essential oil and stir well.
8. Pour the mixture into jar containers.
9. Let the mixture harden.
10. Enjoy your very own homemade floral solid perfume!

Sweet Vanilla Scented Perfume

Prep Time: 5 minutes
Cook Time: 0 minutes
Ready In: 1 week
Servings: approximately 1 perfume bottle

Ingredients:

Sandalwood essential oil (10 drops)

Vanilla essential oil (29 drops)

Jojoba oil (11 ml)

Directions:

1. Using a dropper put the essential oils in a glass bottle. (Glass bottle can be colored or clear.)
2. Close the lid of the bottle and shake the mixture.
3. Add the jojoba oil after shaking the first mixture.

4. Once again close the lid and shake the bottle so that the mixture mixes very well.
5. Let the mixture settle for 1 week in a dark, dry and cool place. Stir the mixture every now and then. Take note that the longer you let the perfume settle and rest, the stronger the scent.
6. Try out the perfume you have created. Shake the bottle well before using the perfume. Rub it on your wrist and neck. Check for any allergic reactions upon the application of the perfume to make sure it is safe on the skin.
7. Enjoy your very own homemade floral perfume!

Ylang ylang and lavender Scented Perfume

Prep Time: 5 minutes
Cook Time: 0 minutes
Ready In: 1 week
Servings: approximately 1 perfume bottle

Ingredients:

Lavender essential oil (9 drops)
Ylang ylang essential oil (10 drops)
Jojoba oil (10 ml)

Directions:

1. Using a dropper put the essential oils in a glass bottle. (Glass bottle can be colored or clear.)
2. Close the lid of the bottle and shake the mixture.
3. Add the jojoba oil after shaking the first mixture.
4. Once again close the lid and shake the bottle so that the mixture mixes very well.
5. Let the mixture settle for 1 week in a dark, dry and cool place. Stir the mixture every now and then. Take note that the longer you let the perfume settle and rest, the stronger the scent.
6. Try out the perfume you have created. Shake the bottle well before using the perfume. Rub it on your

wrist and neck. Check for any allergic reactions upon the application of the perfume to make sure it is safe on the skin.

7. Enjoy your very own homemade floral perfume!

Walk In the Garden Floral Perfume

Prep Time: 5 minutes
Cook Time: 0 minutes
Ready In: 48 hours
Servings: approximately 1 perfume bottle

Ingredients:

Lavender essential oil (9 drops)
Cedar-wood essential oil (6 drops)
Clove essential oil (15 drops)
Sweet almond oil (2 tablespoons)
Distilled water (2 ½ tablespoons)
Vodka (6 tablespoons)

Directions:

1. Using a dropper put the sweet almond in a glass bottle. (Glass bottle can be colored or clear.)
2. Add the essential oils.
3. Shake the bottle for mixing of the liquids.
4. Add the vodka.

5. Close the lid of the bottle and shake
    for several minutes so that everything
    blends well.
6. Let the mixture settle for 48 hours in
    a dark, dry and cool place. Stir the
    mixture every now and then. Take
    note that the more hours you let the
    perfume settle and rest, the stronger
    the scent. So it depends on how long
    you would want the perfume to sleep.
7. Try out the perfume you have
    created. Shake the bottle well before
    using the perfume. Rub it on your
    wrist and neck. Check for any allergic
    reactions upon the application of the
    perfume to make sure it is safe on the
    skin.
8. Enjoy your very own homemade
    floral perfume!

Cypress And Rosemary Scented Perfume

Prep Time: 5 minutes
Cook Time: 0 minutes
Ready In: 12-15 hours
Servings: approximately 1 perfume bottle

Ingredients:

3 tablespoons of either ethyl alcohol or vodka

Cypress essential oil (10 drops)

Rosemary essential oil (10 drops)

Hypericum perforatum essential oil (5 drops)

Distilled water (2 cups)

Directions:

1. In a small glass jar, mix all the essential oils together with the alcohol.
2. Add some amount of distilled water into the mixture.
3. Transfer it into a glass bottle (colored or clear will do).
4. Shake the bottle to make sure the oils, alcohol and water blend together well.
5. Let the mixture settle for 12 to 15 hours in a dark, dry and cool place. Shake the bottle every now and then. Take note that the more hours you let the perfume settle and rest, the stronger the scent.

6. Try out the perfume you have created.
   Shake the bottle well before using the
   perfume. Rub it on your wrist and neck.
   Check for any allergic reactions upon the
   application of the perfume to make sure it
   is safe on the skin.
7. Enjoy your very own homemade floral
   perfume!

Chamomile And Valerian Scented Perfume

Prep Time: 5 minutes
Cook Time: 0 minutes
Ready In: 15 hours
Servings: approximately 1 perfume bottle

Ingredients:

3 tablespoons of either ethyl alcohol or vodka

Chamomile essential oil (10 drops)

Valerian essential oil (10 to 12 drops)

Lavender essential oil (5 drops)

Distilled water (2 cups)

Directions:

1. In a small glass jar, mix all the essential oils
   together with the alcohol.

2. Add some amount of distilled water into the mixture.

3. Transfer it into a glass bottle (colored or clear will do).

4. Shake the bottle to make sure the oils, alcohol and water blend together well.

5. Let the mixture settle for 15 hours in a dark, dry and cool place. Shake the bottle every now and then. Take note that the more hours you let the perfume settle and rest, the stronger the scent.

6. Try out the perfume you have created. Shake the bottle well before using the perfume. Rub it on your wrist and neck. Check for any allergic reactions upon the application of the perfume to make sure it is safe on the skin.

7. Enjoy your very own homemade floral perfume!

Cassis And Bergamot Scented Perfume

Prep Time: 5 minutes
Cook Time: 0 minutes
Ready In: 12-15 hours
Servings: approximately 1 perfume bottle

Ingredients:

    3 tablespoons of either ethyl alcohol or vodka
    Bergamot essential oil (10 drops)
    Cassis essential oil (10 drops
    Sandalwood essential oil (5 drops)
    Distilled water (2 cups)

Directions:

1. In a small glass jar, mix all the essential oils together with the alcohol.
2. Add some amount of distilled water into the mixture.
3. Transfer it into a glass bottle (colored or clear will do).
4. Shake the bottle to make sure the oils, alcohol and water blend together well.
5. Let the mixture settle for 12 to 15 hours in a dark, dry and cool place. Shake the bottle every now and then. Take note that the more hours you let the perfume settle and rest, the stronger the scent.
6. Try out the perfume you have created. Shake the bottle well before using the perfume. Rub it on your wrist and neck. Check for any allergic reactions upon the application of the perfume to make sure it is safe on the skin.

7. Enjoy your very own homemade floral perfume!

43

Musk, Sandalwood And Frankincense Scented Perfume

Prep Time: 5 minutes
Cook Time: 0 minutes
Ready In: 12-15 hours
Servings: approximately 1 perfume bottle

Ingredients:

3 teaspoons of jojoba oil

Musk essential oil (4-5 drops)

Sandalwood essential oil (4 drops)

Frankincense essential oil (3 drops)

Directions:

1. In a small glass jar, mix all the essential oils together with the jojoba oil.

2. Transfer it into a glass bottle (colored or clear will do).

3. Shake the bottle to make sure the oils blend together well.

4. Let the mixture settle for 12 to 15 hours in a dark, dry and cool place. Shake the bottle every now and then. Take note that the more hours you let the perfume settle and rest, the stronger the scent.

5. Try out the perfume you have created. Shake the bottle well before using the perfume. Rub it on your wrist and neck. Check for any allergic reactions upon the application of the perfume to make sure it is safe on the skin.

6. Enjoy your very own homemade floral perfume!

Assorted Essential Oils Scented Perfume

Prep Time: 5 minutes
Cook Time: 0 minutes
Ready In: 10 hours
Servings: approximately 1 perfume bottle

Ingredients:

> Ethyl Alcohol (50 ml)
> Rosemary Essential Oil (30 drops)
> Lemon Essential Oil (12 drops)
> Rose Essential Oil (5 drops)
> Neroil Essential Oil (5 drops)
> Sage Essential Oil (2 drops)
> Mint Essential Oil (2 drops)

Directions:

1. In a small glass jar, mix all the essential oils together with the alcohol.
2. Transfer it into a glass bottle (colored or clear will do).
3. Shake the bottle to make sure the oils and alcohol blend together well.
4. Let the mixture settle for 10 hours in a dark, dry and cool place. Shake the bottle every now and then. Take note that the more hours you let the perfume settle and rest, the stronger the scent.
5. Try out the perfume you have created. Shake the bottle well before using the perfume. Rub it on your wrist and neck. Check for any allergic reactions upon the application of the perfume to make sure it is safe on the skin.

6.   Enjoy your very own homemade floral perfume!

Lavender Scented Perfume

Prep Time: 5 minutes
 Cook Time: 0 minutes
Ready In: 48 hours
Servings: approximately 1 perfume bottle

Ingredients:

Lavender flowers (2 cups)

Boiling water (2 pints)

Vodka (2 tablespoons)

Directions:

1.   Put the two cups of lavender flowers in a container which is heatproof.
2.   Pour in the boiling water.
3.   Add the vodka.
4.   Stir the mixture very well.
5.   Cover the container.
6.   Let the mixture settle for 48 hours in a dark, dry and cool place. Stir the mixture every now and then. Take note that the more hours you let the perfume settle and rest, the stronger the scent.
7.   Strain the liquid using a non-metal strain.
8.   Extract the maximum fragrance of the lavender flowers by pressing them against the sides.
9.   Add more alcohol.
10. Pour the liquid into a glass bottle (colored or clear).

11. Try out the perfume you have created. Shake the
     bottle well before using the perfume. Rub it on your
     wrist and neck. Check for any allergic reactions
     upon the application of the perfume to make sure it
     is safe on the skin.

12. Enjoy your very own homemade floral perfume!

Lilac Scented Perfume

Prep Time: 5 minutes
Cook Time: 0 minutes
Ready In: At least 48 hours
Servings: approximately 1 perfume bottle

Ingredients:

> Lilac flowers (2 cups)
> Boiling water (2 pints)
> Vodka (2 tablespoons)
> Glycerin

Directions:

1. Put the two cups of lilac flowers in a
   container which is heatproof and
   flameproof.
2. Pour in the boiling water.
3. Add the vodka and 2 drops of glycerin.
4. Stir the mixture very well.
5. Cover the container.
6. Let the mixture settle for 48 hours in a dark,
   dry and cool place. Stir the mixture every
   now and then. Take note that the more

hours you let the perfume settle and rest, the stronger the scent.

7. Strain the liquid using a non-metal strain. Cheesecloth will do.
8. Extract the maximum fragrance of the lilac flowers by pressing them against the sides.
9. Add a little more vodka.
10. Pour the liquid into a glass bottle (colored or clear).
11. Try out the perfume you have created. Shake the bottle well before using the perfume.
Rub it on your wrist and neck. Check for any allergic reactions upon the application of the perfume to make sure it is safe on the skin.
12. Enjoy your very own homemade floral perfume!

Rose Scented Perfume

Prep Time: 5 minutes

Cook Time: 0 minutes

Ready In: 2-3 weeks

Servings: approximately 1 perfume bottle

Ingredients:

Rose essential oil (30 drops)

Vodka (3 ounces)

Directions:

1. On a container, mix the essential oil to the vodka.
2. Gently shake the container to mix the oil and alcohol.
3. Let the mixture age for 2 to 3 weeks, in a dark, dry and cool place. Take note that the longer you let the perfume age and rest, the stronger the scent will be so it depends on how long you want the perfume to sleep.
4. After letting the mixture settle, cool it for a short while.
5. Filter the mixture using a coffee filter and a funnel.
6. Let the perfume settle.
7. Chill and filter the mixture again if there are still traces of oil which is isn't dissolved.
8. Try out the perfume you have created. Shake the bottle well before using the perfume. Rub it on your wrist and neck. Check for any

allergic reactions upon the application of the
perfume to make sure it is safe on the skin.

9.   Enjoy your very own homemade floral
perfume!

Orange Blossoms Scented Perfume

Prep Time: 5 minutes
Cook Time: 0 minutes
Ready In: 24 hours
Servings: approximately 1 perfume bottle

Ingredients:

Orange blossoms (2 cups)

Boiling water (2 pints)

Vodka (2 tablespoons)

Directions:

1.   Put the two cups of orange blossoms in a
container which is heatproof.
2.   Pour in the boiling water.
3.   Add the vodka.
4.   Stir the mixture very well.
5.   Cover the container.
6.   Let the mixture settle for 24 hours in a dark,
dry and cool place. Stir the mixture every now
and then. Take note of the fact that that the
more hours you let the perfume settle and rest,
the stronger the scent.

7. Strain the liquid using a non-metal strain.

8. Extract the maximum fragrance of the orange blossoms by pressing them against the sides.

9. Pour the liquid into a glass bottle (colored or clear).

10. Try out the perfume you have created. Shake the bottle well before using the perfume. Rub it on your wrist and neck. Check for any allergic reactions upon the application of the perfume to make sure it is safe on the skin.

11. Enjoy your very own homemade floral perfume!

Orange and Cinnamon Scented Perfume

Prep Time: 5 minutes
Cook Time: 0 minutes
Ready In: 2 to 6 weeks
Servings: approximately 1 perfume bottle

Ingredients:

Organic Cardamom pods (25 pieces whole)
Organic Vanilla Bean (1 piece)
Vodka (8 ounces)
Cinnamon sticks (1 piece)
Organic Cloves (15 pieces)
Organic zest orange peel (1 piece)

Directions:

1. Cut the vanilla bean into small pieces.

2. Using a mortar and pestle, crush all the spices.

3. Mix the crushed spices with the vanilla bean, vodka and orange peel in a glass jar.
4. Close the glass jar.
5. Let the mixture settle for 2-6 weeks in a dark, dry and cool place. Stir the mixture every now and then, say once or more daily. Take note of the fact that that the more hours you let the perfume settle and rest, the stronger the scent.
6. Strain the liquid using a non-metal strain.
7. Pour the liquid into a glass bottle (colored or clear).
8. Try out the perfume you have created. Shake the bottle well before using the perfume. Rub it on your wrist and neck. Check for any allergic reactions upon the application of the perfume to make sure it is safe on the skin.
9. Enjoy your very own homemade floral perfume!

Rose, Chamomile and Lavender Scented Perfume

Prep Time: 5 minutes
Cook Time: 0 minutes
Ready In: 48 hours
Servings: approximately 1 small perfume bottle

Ingredients:

Organic jojoba oil (1 teaspoon)

Lemon essential oil (5 drops)

Juniper berry essential oil (5 drops)

Organic sage essential oil (5 drops)

Organic peppermint essential oil (13 drops)

Organic rosemary essential oil (13 drops)

Directions:

1. Using a dropper, drip the essential oils into a glass bottle (colored or clear glass bottle will do).
2. Close the bottle.
3. Shake the bottle to mix all the essential oils.
4. Drip the jojoba oil.
5. Shake the bottle once again to mix the oils.
6. Let the mixture settle for 24 hours, in a dark, dry and cool place. Shake the bottle every now and then. Take note of the fact that that the more hours you let the perfume settle and rest, the stronger the scent.

7.   Try out the perfume you have created. Shake the
     bottle well before using the perfume. Rub it on
     your wrist and neck. Check for any allergic
     reactions upon the application of the perfume to
     make sure it is safe on the skin.
8.   Enjoy your very own homemade floral perfume!

Foresty Scented Perfume

Prep Time: 5 minutes

Cook Time: 0 minutes

Ready In: 48 hours

Servings: approximately 1 small perfume bottle

Ingredients:

   Organic jojoba oil (1 teaspoon)
   Bergamot essential oil (1 drop)
   Cedarwood essential oil (2 drops)
    Spruce essential oil (4 drops)
   Organic Fir needle essential oil (2 drops)
   Organic vetiver essential oil (1 drop)

Directions:

1.   Using a dropper, drip the essential oils into a
     glass bottle (colored or clear glass bottle will
     do).
2.   Close the bottle.
3.   Shake the bottle to mix all the essential oils.
4.   Drip the jojoba oil.
5.   Shake the bottle once again to mix the oils.
6.   Let the mixture settle for 48 hours, in a dark,
     dry and cool place. Shake the bottle every now

and then. Take note of the fact that that the more hours you let the perfume settle and rest, the stronger the scent.

7. Try out the perfume you have created. Shake the bottle well before using the perfume. Rub it on your wrist and neck. Check for any allergic reactions upon the application of the perfume to make sure it is safe on the skin.

8. Enjoy your very own homemade floral perfume!

Summer Scent Perfume

Prep Time: 5 minutes
Cook Time: 0 minutes
Ready In: 48 hours
Servings: approximately 1 small perfume bottle

Ingredients:

Organic jojoba oil (1 teaspoon)

Cardamom essential oil (4 drops)

Organic lavender essential oil (10 drops)

Organic Cedarwood essential oil (1 drop)

Organic chamomile essential oil (5 drops)

Organic Rose essential oil (1 drop)

Directions:

1.   Using a dropper, drip the essential oils into
     a glass bottle (colored or clear glass bottle
     will do).
2.   Close the bottle.
3.   Shake the bottle to mix all the essential oils.
4.   Drip the jojoba oil.
5.   Shake the bottle once again to mix the oils.
6.   Let the mixture settle for 48 hours, in a
     dark, dry and cool place. Shake the bottle
     every now and then. Take note of the fact
     that that the more hours you let the
     perfume settle and rest, the stronger the
     scent.
7.   Try out the perfume you have created.
     Shake the bottle well before using the
     perfume. Rub it on your wrist and neck.
     Check for any allergic reactions upon the
     application of the perfume to make sure it is
     safe on the skin.
8.   Enjoy your very own homemade floral
     perfume!

Sweet Floral Scent Perfume

Prep Time: 5 minutes
Cook Time: 0 minutes
Ready In: 48 hours
Servings: approximately 1 small perfume bottle

Ingredients:

Organic jojoba oil (2 tablespoons)
Patchouli oil (4 drops)
Organic geranium essential oil (12 drops)
Organic bergamot essential oil (3 drops)
Organic jasmine essential oil (8 drops)
Organic neroli essential oil (2 drops)
Organic Rose essential oil (8 drops)

Directions:

1. Using a dropper, drip the essential oils into a glass bottle (colored or clear glass bottle will do).
2. Close the bottle.
3. Shake the bottle to mix all the essential oils.
4. Add the jojoba oil to the mixture.
5. Shake the bottle once again to mix the oils.
6. Let the mixture settle for 48 hours, in a dark, dry and cool place. Shake the bottle every now and then. Take note of the fact that that the more hours you let the perfume settle and rest, the stronger the scent.
7. Try out the perfume you have created. Shake the bottle well before using the perfume. Rub it on your wrist and neck. Check for any allergic reactions upon the application of the perfume to make sure it is safe on the skin.

8.   Enjoy your very own homemade floral perfume!

Gorgeous Floral Scented Perfume
Prep Time: 5 minutes
Cook Time: 0 minutes
Ready In: 3 days
Servings: approximately 1 small perfume bottle

Ingredients:

Sandalwood essential oil (3 drops)

Rose essential oil (2 drops)

Vanilla essential oil (5 drops)

Jasmine essential oil (2 drops)

Bergamot essential oil (6 drops)

Grapeseed oil (half ounce)

Directions:

1   Using a dropper, drip the essential oils into a glass bottle (colored or clear glass bottle will do).
2   Close the bottle.
3   Shake the bottle to mix all the essential oils.
4   Add the grapeseed oil to the mixture.
5   Shake the bottle once again to mix the oils.
6   Let the mixture settle for 3 days, in a dark, dry and cool place. Shake the bottle every now and then. Take note of the fact that that the more hours you

let the perfume settle and rest, the stronger the scent.

7   Try out the perfume you have created. Shake the bottle well before using the perfume. Rub it on your wrist and neck. Check for any allergic reactions upon the application of the perfume to make sure it is safe on the skin.

8   Enjoy your very own homemade floral perfume!

MIXED PERFUME RECIPES

Sweet Flowery Perfume Recipe

Prep Time: 15 minutes
Cook Time: 0 minutes
Ready In: 24 hours
Servings: 1 small perfume bottle

Ingredients:

1 cup distilled water

10 drops organic lavender essential oil

5 drops organic chamomile essential oil

4 drops organic cardamom essential oil

1 drop organic cedar wood essential oil

1 drop organic geranium (rose) essential oil

1 tsp organic jojoba oil

Directions:

1. Drip all the essential oils into a glass bottle.

2. Roll the bottle between your palms to evenly mix the oil

3. Add jojoba oil and mix again.

4   Add distilled water

5   Let all the essential oil seep together

for about 24 hours

Your perfume is ready. Now apply on wrists or behind the
ears for a fresh summery smell!

Refreshing Woody Body Mist

Prep Time: 20 minutes
Cook Time: 0 minutes
Ready In: 24 hours
Servings: 1 small perfume bottle

Ingredients:

30 ml distilled water

10 ml rose water

2 tsp vanilla extract

1 tsp vodka

1tbsp vegetable glycerin

6 tbsp coconut oil

6 drops grapefruit essential oil

Directions:

1. Fill your spray bottle with lukewarm distilled and rose water
2. Mix the vanilla extract
3. Add vegetable glycerin
4. Add coconut oil
5. Now add the essential oil
6. Give the bottle a good shake
7. Let it rest for 24 hours

Your perfume is ready. Now apply on wrists or behind the ears for a refreshing citrusy smell.

Refreshing Citrus Mist

Prep Time: 20 minutes
Cook Time: 0 minutes
Ready In: 24 hours
Servings: 1 small perfume bottle

Ingredients:

30 ml distilled water
10 ml rose water

2 tsp vanilla extract

1 tsp vodka

1tbsp vegetable glycerin

1 tbsp coconut oil

5 drops grapefruit essential oil

Directions:

1. Fill your spray bottle with lukewarm distilled and rose water
2. Mix the vanilla extract
3. Add vegetable glycerin
4. Add coconut oil
5. Now add the essential oil
6. Give the bottle a good shake
7. Let it rest for 24 hours

Your perfume is ready. Now apply on wrists or behind the ears for a refreshing citrusy smell.

Refreshing Lavender And Vanilla Mist

Prep Time: 20 minutes once and 20 minutes again after first session
Cook Time: 0 minutes
Ready In: 8 weeks
Servings: 1 small perfume bottle

Ingredients:

¼ glass vodka
2 tsp glycerin
1 cup dried lavender flower
2 crushed vanilla beans
10 drops lavender essential oil
8 drops vanilla extract

Directions:

1. Take the crushed beans along with the dried lavender flowers and put in a small jar

2. Mix the vodka in

3. Close the lid and let it sit for about one week

4. After one week open the jar and strain the extract

5. Now add the lavender essential oil, vanilla extract and glycerin

6. Stir the mixture

7.   Close the lid again and let the mixture sit for about 3 to 4 weeks

8. Take out the liquid and empty it into a glass bottle

Your wonderful lavender and vanilla perfume is ready. It will remind you of fresh summery days, so go out and have some fun!

Flowery Scent

Prep Time: 10 minutes
Cook Time: 0 minutes
Ready In: 3 days
Servings: 1 small perfume bottle

Ingredients:

  2 drops jasmine essential oil

  6 drops bergamot essential oil

  3 drops sandalwood essential oil

  5 drops vanilla extract

  2 drops Rose essential oils

Directions:

1. Mix all the essential oils together
2. Now add the vanilla extract
3. Slowly shake the bottle
4. Let the mixture seep together for 3 days

Get ready to smell gorgeous. This perfume will help you smell like a flower and attract potential suitors☺.

Fresh Peppermint And Vanilla Perfume

Prep Time: 10 minutes
Cook Time: 0 minutes
Ready In: 2 days
Servings: 1 small perfume bottle

Ingredients:

10 drops vanilla essential oil

2   drops peppermint essential oil

9drops lavender essential oil

Directions:

1. Mix all the essential oils together

2. Slowly shake the bottle

3. Let the mixture seep together for 3 days

Get ready to smell fresh and flowery.

Sandalwood And Cassis Perfume

Prep Time: 10 minutes
Cook Time: 0 minutes
Ready In: 2 days
Servings: 1 small perfume bottle

Ingredients:

5 drops bergamot essential oil

3 drops sandalwood essential oil

5 drops cassis essential oil

1 cup distilled water

5 tsp vodka

Directions:

1. Mix all the essential oils together
2. Slowly shake the bottle
3. Now slowly stir in the vodka
4. Add distilled water
5. Let the mixture seep for 2 days

Your refreshing sandalwood and cassis perfume is ready.

Relaxing Chamomile and Jasmine Perfume

Prep Time: 10 minutes
Cook Time: 0 minutes
Ready In: 1 day
Servings: 1 small perfume bottle

Ingredients:

2 cups distilled water

3 tbsp vodka

5 drops lavender essential oil

10 drops chamomile essential oil

10 drops valerian essential oil

Directions:

1) Mix all the essential oils together

2) Slowly shake the bottle

3) Now slowly stir in the vodka

4) Add distilled water

5) Let the mixture seep for about a day

Your relaxing jasmine and chamomile perfume is ready.

Refreshing Lemon Grass and Geranium Perfume

Prep Time: 15 minutes
Cook Time: 0 minutes
Ready In: 2 days
Servings: 1 perfume bottle

Ingredients:

½ ounce jojoba essential oil

2 ounces vodka

1 ounce distilled water

4 drops Vanilla essential oil

4 drops lemongrass essential oil

5 drops jasmine essential oil

10 drops lavender essential oil

4 drops geranium essential oil

Directions:

1) Mix all the essential oils together

2) Slowly shake the bottle

3) Now slowly stir in the vodka

4) Add distilled water

5) Let the mixture seep for about a day

Your relaxing jasmine and chamomile perfume is ready

Refreshing Oriental Scent

Prep Time: 15 minutes
Cook Time: 0 minutes
Ready In: 12 hours
Servings: 1 perfume bottle

Ingredients:

4 drops sandalwood essential oil

4 drops musk essential oil

3 drops cardamom essential oil

2 tsp jojoba oil

Directions:

1) Mix all the essential oils together

2) Slowly shake the bottle

3) Add distilled water

4) Let the mixture seep for about 12 hours

This lovely scent will transport you to the beautiful smelling gardens of the orient

SCENTED WATERS

Another excellent way of perfuming the body, scented water can either be splashed on having a cool bath or put in a diffuser bottle and sprayed on the body. To make scented water, infuse distilled water with various ingredients. Only fresh ingredients should be used for scented waters because the juicier the better. Here are some ideas to get you started:

Orange Water

(Lemon water is another variant, substitute lemon peel for orange peel in this recipe).

Ingredients:

Vodka (1/2 cup)

Distilled water (3 cups)

Orange peel chopped into pieces (1/2 cup)

Directions:

1. Place the vodka and orange peel a glass measuring cup. Allow to sit for one day.
2. Use a wooden spoon to mash and then add the distilled water.
3. Allow to sit one week while mixing and mashing once a day.
4. Strain the water into a bottle
5. Use the water to perfume your body.

Rose Water

Ingredients:

Vodka (1/2 cup)

Distilled water (3 cups)

Fresh rose petals (1/2 cup)

Directions

1. Place the vodka and rose petals in a glass measuring cup. Allow to sit one day.
2. Use a wooden spoon to mash and then add the distilled water.
3. Allow to sit one week while mixing and mashing once a day.
4. Strain the water into a bottle.
5. Use the water to perfume your body.

Lavender Water

Ingredients:

Vodka (1/2 cup)

Distilled water (3 cups)

Fresh lavender flowers (1/2 cup)

Directions:

1. Place the vodka and lavender in a glass measuring cup and allow to sit one day.
2. Use a wooden spoon to mash and then add the distilled water.
3. Allow to sit one week while mixing and mashing once a day.
4. Strain the water into a bottle use,
5. Use the water to perfume your body.

Rosemary Water

(Try making rosemary lemon water as well. these two fragrances when mixed is extremely refreshing).

Ingredients:

Vodka (1/2 cup)

Distilled water (3 cups)

Chopped fresh rosemary (1/2 cup)

Directions:

1. Place the vodka and rosemary in a glass measuring cup. Allow to sit for one day.
2. Use a wooden spoon to mash and then add the distilled water.
3. Allow to sit one week while mixing and mashing once a day.
4. Strain the water into a bottle
5. Use the water to perfume your body.

The End